DISCLAIMER

This book is not a substitute for professional medical diagnosis or treatment. Please consult with your doctor, pharmacist or health authority before trying any treatment suggested in this book.

Acne

Acne has affected most of my family for a considerable time. A few years ago, I decided to look for an alternative approach to treat this annoying problem.

It was time to look at more natural ways to get rid of acne!

All treatments, have been researched and applied to either myself or my family.

I hope you enjoy trying out the different treatments to finally get rid of your acne.

Caution!

If you find, that any treatment in this book   has an adverse effect.. Stop the treatment immediately and try another tip in the book.

Advice

You may find, that some remedies are more suitable than others.

Read through all the tips and start with the most practical remedy first.

To get the most out of this book, it's wise to follow the daily schedule that is recommended for each tip.

Index

Index

(Continued)

Tip 1

Aloe Vera

There are two types of Aloe Vera you can use. Buy the gel in pure form or if you have the Aloe Vera plant squeeze the sap from the leaves, into a bowl. It's much easier to buy the gel from a drugstore.

- Apply the gel topically 2-3 times daily.

- There is a slight odor but it fades quickly

Aloe does tighten the skin a little, even oily skin dries out. So applying Jojoba cream 20 minutes after the initial treatment helps the skin hold in moisture.

Tip 2

Aloe Vera and Milk Thistle

This is a different approach. Using Aloe Vera juice instead of the gel.

 Consume approximately 10oz of Aloe Vera juice per day, and take 250mg of Milk Thistle with each meal.

Milk Thistle helps the liver eliminate toxins from the body.

You may find you're bowel movements become more regular.

Tip 3

Apple Cider Vinegar

The best ACV to purchase is organic. You can apply the ACV Topically to the face. I recommend that you test out a small are of your skin first!

Start by drinking 2 teaspoons 3 times a day, gradually building up to 2 tablespoons and applying it topically each night using a cotton ball.

Another alternative is drinking organic ACV with Manuka honey in hot water 3x daily is a more pleasant way to consume Apple Cider Vinegar.

WARNING: DO NOT apply apple cider vinegar straight to your face before making sure you're not allergic to it.

Tip 4

Aspirin and Manuka Honey Face Mask

This face mask is a must for all all Acne sufferers, after a few treatments a noticeable difference in your skin should be visible.

What you need to make the face mask is:

- 5 effervescent aspirins (soluble)
- 1 tablespoon of Manuka Honey
- Few drops of water
- Crush the aspirin and mix it with the water
- Add the honey and mix well
- Apply to the face and leave it on for 15 minutes
- Wash off and gently pat dry

Aspirin dries the skin out somewhat, so apply some Jojoba moisturizer to the face once dry.

Tip 5

Aspirin and Calamine Lotion

This amazing face wash leaves your skin cool and calm.

If you can find aspirin powders, that works best, otherwise plain aspirin will do.

- Empty two Aspirin powders into a small bowl.
- Add enough Calamine lotion to make a creamy paste.
- Apply to the face gently in a circular motion.
- Leave it on for 5-10 minutes.
- Gently rinse off.
- Pat-dry the face and apply a good moisturizer.

Tip 6

Apple Cider Vinegar Steam

Add 2 tablespoons of ACV to a pot of boiling water, place a towel over you're head to trap the steam.

Steaming will loosen dirt and oil.

After you have steamed the facial area, soak a cotton ball in some Apple Cider Vinegar, to wipe away the oil and dirt.

Be careful when steaming to prevent any burns.

Tip 7

Baking Soda

(Sodium Bicarbonate)

Combine 2 tablespoons of Baking Soda with some water to make a paste.

Massage the paste around the face using circular motions. Concentrate on the areas with the most scarring.

After about a minute gently rinse off.

Repeat this process once daily.

Tip 8

Carrot & Broccoli Juice

Note: you will need a Juicer to extract the juice from the carrots and Broccoli.

- Use 4-5 organic carrots scraped and washed and a small bunch of Broccoli.

You can also sweeten the drink by adding an apple.

Try and get into a habit of drinking fresh carrot and Broccoli juice daily.

Tip 9

Castor Oil

Castor oil works great in dissolving oil from the pores (Blackheads).

Put a small blob of castor oil in the palm of you're hand.
Gently rub the castor oil into your skin.

- Leave it on for 2-3 minutes.
- Use a hot face-cloth to wipe off.
- Then finally apply a good oil-free moisturizer.

Tip 10

Coconut Oil

This amazing oil works great externally and internally

Its always best to use Virgin Coconut Oil.

Coconut oil is antiviral and antibacterial, and best of all, it's a good fat. Start by consuming 1 tablespoon of oil a day and gradually building up to 3x daily.

After each face wash you can apply Virgin Coconut Oil to the skin as a healing moisturizer.

Tip 11

Cucumber

Cucumber is said to clean the lymphatic system and purify the blood, leaving the skin clearer.

Note: you will need an electric blender.

- In a blender liquify a peeled cucumber.
- Apply the juice to the problem areas.
- Leave to dry.
- Drink 3-4 cups of cucumber juice daily.
- Continue this daily for 10 days.

Tip 12

Egg

Try whisking an egg in a bowl, and slice up a raw potato.

Dip a slice of potato in the bowl with the egg and gently apply it to the affected areas.

Leave it on for 10 minutes, then rinse off.

Do this once in the morning and at night.

Repeat this treatment for 1 week and your skin will feel softer and have a healthy glow.

Tip 13

Epsom Salts

The bacteria that causes acne, does not like a salty environment. Epsom salts are renowned for drawing impurities out of the skin.

Simply measure out 1 tablespoon of Epsom Salts into the wash hand basin, whisk it around with your hands until the salts dissolve.

Splash the salty water over your face for a minute, then pat dry.

If you feel you're skin tightening, use a moisturizer such as Jojoba or Coconut oil.

Tip 14

Essential Oils

This treatment involves three kinds of essential oils. Lavender, Tea tree and Rosemary.

You will also need a small clean spray bottle.

Simply add 2-3 drops of the oils into the bottle and fill up with warm water and give it a good shake.

Spray it on a clean dry face every morning and night, be careful to avoid the eyes.

Store the bottle when not in use in a dark cool place.

Always shake the bottle prior to using.

Tip 15

Evening Primrose Oil

This treatment is more suitable for women, due to the fact that Evening primrose oil has hormone-regulating qualities.

Evening Primrose Oil also has unique anti-inflammatory properties.

The recommended dosage is 1 x 500mg capsule three times daily.

Tip 16

Garlic

Caution garlic does have a burning effect on the skin!

Test on a small area first?

What we found was, it's best to purchase garlic capsules, they are more gentle on the skin.

Gently pierce two or three garlic capsules in a small bowl.

Add a little Manuka Honey and a few drops of warm water.

Apply this mixture to the affected area for 3-4 minutes, then rinse off.

Repeat daily until symptoms clear up.

Tip 17

Green Tea

This remedy works best using a Green Tea teabag.

Place a teabag in a mug of hot water and let it cool so it's just warm.

Take the teabag out of the mug and gently wipe your face with it.

Let the skin dry naturally.

Green Tea can stain the skin slightly, so once dry you can rinse of the residue.

Tip 18

Lemons

Lemon juice is good for killing toxins and also for reducing redness in the skin.

Squeeze the juice out from a lemon, and use a cotton ball to apply to the skin.

You can apply coconut oil once the lemon juice has dried up on the skin.

Always use lemon juice sparingly.

Tip 19

Honey, Nutmeg and Lemon

This is another face-mask treatment.

Put 2 tablespoons of Manuka honey into a small bowl.

Add half a squeezed Lemon and a quarter teaspoon of Nutmeg.

Mix it all together and apply to the affected area.

Try and leave it on for 30 minutes, then wash off.

Continue with this daily until your symptoms clear up.

Tip 20

3% Food Grade Hydrogen peroxide

Caution: It's important to use 3% food grade Hydrogen Peroxide!

This is a very popular way to treat Acne at home.

You can purchase Hydrogen Peroxide from the Internet.
It usually comes in a handy spray bottle, ready for use.

Simply spray on the affected area and leave to dry.

Or you can spray on to a cotton ball then dab it on the skin.

Always avoid the area around the eyes.

Repeat this ritual every morning and night.

Tip 21

Honey and cinnamon paste

This is another effective face mask, that leaves the skin so fresh.

Use 3 parts of honey to part cinnamon powder.

Apply the paste to the skin and leave on for 30 minutes.

It normally takes 2-3 weeks until the symptoms start to clear.

Tip 22

Milk of Magnesia

This is an amazing mask to draw out the impurities and treat acne. You can use this mask once a week or daily for oily skin.

The liquid will dry and harden quickly, so i suggest you wet your face first before applying Milk of Magnesia.

It's best to put the solution on at night before you go to bed.
Simply pour enough on the palm of the hands to cover the area and leave it on for 5-10 minutes, then rinse off.

It works slowly but everyday you will notice the acne getting smaller and smaller.

Tip 23

Ozonated Olive Oil

Ozonated oil was first used by the Germans in WW1, but since Antibiotics have become the main-stay in fighting infections. Ozonated oil or (Activated oxygen) as it's sometimes called lay forgotten.

The oil is rich in oxygen and has a fresh smell.

You can purchase this oil from the Internet. There is also some sites that explain in more detail, of it's many uses.

Generally Ozonated oil comes in a handy tub and should be kept in the refrigerator.

As with all creams, rub a small amount onto the affected area twice daily.

Tip 24

PANTOTHENIC ACID

(Vitamin B5)

High doses of (Vitamin B5) may decrease pore size. Many people are without sufficient quantities of Pantothenic Acid in there bodies.

Start taking the daily recommended allowance, 5 days out of 7.

If you find this remedy suitable, an improvement should be noticeable within a week to a month.

Tip 25

Probiotics

Adding Probiotics to every meal ensures your digestive system stays healthy.

Pro-biotic drinks restore good bacteria to fight infections!

This friendly bacteria helps to heal the digestive system which in turn has an amazing effect on the skin

And it's cheap!

Tip 26

Sea Salt

Fill up your sink up with warm water. Then pour some salt into it. Soak a cotton ball in the salty water and swish it around, making sure its all salty.

Squeeze out the cotton ball and apply it on the acne.

If your face doesn't start to tingle, add more salt to the cotton ball. When your face does start tingling, push down for 3 minutes. After 3 minutes, Don't wash the salt of your face.

Another way to use the salt remedy is to add some sea salt to a wet-paper-towel and apply to the pimples until it stings, if it stings it's working.

Tip 27

Sandalwood and Water

This treatment will help brighten up the face and reduce the size of the pores.

Take a spoonful of sandalwood powder, add a little warm water to it, mixing it into a paste, then apply it to your face.

Once the mask dries up, use a warm wet cloth and wipe off the paste, rinse the face with warm and then cold water several times

Repeat once daily until the skin looks clearer.

Tip 28

Strawberries

According to the Ancient Egyptians, fresh Strawberries help replenish the skin.

You can also mash the Strawberries up, and apply as a face pack.

Wet Strawberry leaves applied to the face topically may also help alleviate the acne.

Another treatment is to crush some Strawberries up and mix them with a little Apple Cider Vinegar to make a face-pack. Let the mixture soak for an hour then strain the pulp.

Apply the face mask every night to the acne.

You can store the remainder in the refrigerator for up-to 2 days.

You should notice a difference within 3- 4 weeks!

Tip 29

Tea Tree Oil

If you suffer from acne cysts which are long lasting and difficult to treat. Tea Tree Oil may be the answer.

You can use the oil undiluted, but if you have sensitive skin, you may need to dilute it first.

After washing your face, apply the Tea Tree Oil with a cotton swab 1-2 times daily.

For people with sensitive skin, a 60/40 ratio mix with Jojoba cream may be more appropriate. Use a q-tip and apply twice daily to blemishes and red spots.

You can also mix the Tea Tree Oil with water. One part oil to 4 parts water, and apply with a cotton swab.

You may see an improvement within as little as two days!

Tip 30

Turmeric

Turmeric is a spice that's widely used in India. It adds color and flavor to foods.

Turmeric is inexpensive to buy. The spice can be bought loose or in capsule form (if you don't like the taste).

Add 1-2 teaspoons in a glass of warm water, stir well and drink Immediately. Do this 3x daily.

Sometimes the contents settle to the bottom of the glass, so keep stirring.

Turmeric capsules can also be purchased, from most good health stores.

Take 2 capsules 3x daily until your symptoms clear up. There after, you can change to a lower maintenance dose

Tip 31

Urine Therapy

Don't let this treatment put you off!

Human urine contains waste antibodies and it's sterile. It's not as bad as it seems, once dry there's virtually no smell.

It's always best to use fresh urine!

Splash the area to be treated with warm water. Then using your own fresh urine, apply first thing in the morning, soak a cotton ball and then apply the warm urine to the affected area liberally

Leave it on for 15 minutes or until it dries. Then wash off thoroughly.

You'll be amazed how effective this treatment works.

Tip 32

Water

The benefits of drinking 8 glasses of water a day are well documented. Drinking herbal tea also counts towards your 8 glasses.

You can also use ice and steam to treat your acne.

Placing an ice cube on the affected area for 30 seconds 3 times daily will help cool the skin.

Steam your face by boiling water in a pan and place your face over it. Trap the steam with a towel over your head. Don't steam for longer than 10 minutes..After the steam opens the pores splash cold water on your face to close the pores.

Continue this regime for 2-3 weeks or until the acne clears up.

Tip 33

Witch Hazel

Witch Hazel comes in a nice liquid form.

It's quite good for clearing up redness around the face.

Soak a cotton ball with the solution and apply every night after washing your face.

Witch hazel can sting a little, when applied to acne.

You may feel it dries the skin out a little so apply some Jojoba cream, or Virgin Coconut oil to give the skin a nice glow.

You will notice the face feels smooth and fresh.

Tip 34

Natural Yogurt

Natural yogurt reduces swelling and redness it also calms the skin and shrinks pores.

Make sure the yogurt you purchase contains live cultures.

Apply enough natural yogurt to the area, so it's about ¼ to ½ inch thick. Don't spread it to thickly as it will slide down your face.

Leave the yogurt on for up to an hour, until it dries.

You can also add some Manuka honey to the yogurt, mix well then apply as above.

Natural yogurt is gentle enough to use everyday.

Tip 35

Zinc Oxide

(For White Heads)

This is a very inexpensive treatment, most good drug stores will stock Zinc Oxide cream.

Apply the cream topically to the white heads, Twice daily..

The cream does tingle a little when applied.

Bonus

Banana Skin

Nobody knows why banana skin works, but it is very effective.

It clears the skin of blemishes and has good nourishing qualities.

Steam your face first, to open up the pores.

Peel back the skin from a banana.

Use the inside of the skin and gently rub over the acne.

Leave it to dry for 30 minutes, then rinse.

Bonus

Infrared

Note: you will need a mall hand held Infrared device.

Infrared has all the benefits of sunlight without the harmful UV rays.

This kind of light can penetrate a few centimeters into the body, which has an amazing healing effect.

Simply shine the light on to the acne for a few minutes a day.

Caution: Infrared light is invisible to the naked eye, be careful not to shine the light into the eyes.

Bonus

Colloidal Silver

Colloidal Silver can be purchased online and it's not expensive.

Normally it comes in a handy spray bottle.

Silver is a very effective natural antibiotic.

Simply spray the solution on to the acne twice daily and leave to dry naturally.

Bonus

Sillicea

Sillicea is a homeopathic remedy that is popular in India.

It's good for cystic acne and works well drying out small infections.

Sillicea is also good for acne scars.

Take two small tablets 3 times daily until your symptoms improve then reduce the dosage, to 1 tablet 3 x daily.

Sillicea, also known as (sillica,) can be made from grinding semi-quartz stone into a fine powder. Then mixed with water.

Sillicea is available to buy online or in any good homeopathic store.

Bonus

Oil of Oregano

Oregano oil is Antiviral and has Antibiotic properties.

You can buy the oil in a liquid form and also in capsules.

A combination of both treatments is advised.

Take 1 capsule 3 x daily.

Apply some oil to a cotton swab and apply to the affected area.

Photo Credit

Thanks to Robert & Reece
who I love dearly.